The Beginner's Guide to Intermittent Fasting

A Step-by-Step Plan to Lose Weight, Improve Your Health, and Live Longer

Betty B. Burton

Table of Contents

Introduction

Have you ever looked in the mirror and felt a twinge of frustration, maybe even despair? Perhaps you've tried countless diets and exercise routines, only to find yourself stuck in a cycle of hope and disappointment. I've been there too, and I understand that feeling all too well.

In a world saturated with weight loss promises and health fads, it's easy to become skeptical and weary. You may have come across countless books claiming to hold the secret to a healthier, happier life. But here's the truth: this book is different.

"The Beginner's Guide to Intermittent Fasting: A Step-by-Step Plan to Lose Weight, Improve Your Health, and Live Longer" is not just another promise; it's a roadmap to a transformation that transcends the number on the scale. It's a journey towards a better, more vibrant you, and I'm inviting you to embark on this transformative path with me.

Let's face it, we're all searching for something more, something that goes beyond mere physical appearance. We want the energy to play with our children, the vitality to pursue our passions, and the assurance of a long and healthy life. We want to break free from the shackles of cravings and unhealthy eating habits that have held us captive for far too long.

This book is about regaining control, not just of your body but of your life. It's about understanding the science of intermittent fasting, harnessing its power, and crafting a lifestyle that promotes your best self. It's a path to shedding those extra pounds, boosting your confidence, and discovering a sense of empowerment you may have long forgotten.

But it's not just about the destination; it's about the journey. It's about the small victories, the "aha" moments, and the newfound self-respect that will accompany you along the way. It's about the supportive community you'll find within these pages, and the real-life stories of individuals who have transformed their lives through the principles shared in this book.

If you've ever yearned for a brighter, healthier future, you're not alone. And if you're looking for a way to reclaim your life from the clutches of poor health and unwanted weight, you've come to the right place.

Chapter 1

Getting Started with Intermittent Fasting

Setting Clear Goals

Picture this: You wake up one day, look in the mirror, and decide that it's time for a change. You're ready to shed those extra pounds, boost your energy, and improve your health. Intermittent fasting is your ticket to achieving these goals, but to succeed, you need a roadmap. That's where setting clear and meaningful goals comes into play. In this chapter, we'll not only show you how to set achievable goals but also guide you on how to make them a reality.

Introduction:

Intermittent fasting offers a path to a healthier and more vibrant you. It's not just another diet fad; it's a lifestyle shift that can transform your relationship with food, your body, and your overall well-being. But before you dive headfirst into this journey, it's crucial to have a clear destination in mind.

Why Setting Clear Goals Matters:

Imagine setting off on a road trip without a destination. You might drive aimlessly, make wrong turns, and ultimately feel lost and frustrated. The same applies to your intermittent fasting journey. Setting clear goals gives you direction, purpose, and a vision of what you want to achieve. It's the compass that guides you through the challenges and temptations you'll encounter along the way.

The Keys to Effective Goal Setting:

1. Specificity: Vague goals like "I want to lose weight" won't cut it. Get specific. Define how much weight you want to lose, by when, and what other health improvements you seek.

2. Realistic and Sustainable: Set goals that are challenging but attainable. Aiming to lose 50 pounds in a month is neither realistic nor healthy. Focus on gradual, sustainable changes.

3. Measurable: Your goals should be quantifiable. This way, you can track your progress and celebrate your achievements. Use numbers, like "I want to lose 15 pounds" or "I want to reduce my fasting blood sugar level by 20 points."

4. Time-Bound: Assign a timeframe to your goals. For instance, "I aim to lose 15 pounds in the next three months." Having a deadline creates a sense of urgency and commitment.

5. Positive and Motivating: Frame your goals in a positive light. Instead of saying, "I want to stop overeating," say, "I want to make healthier food choices to nourish my body."

6. Authentic and Genuine: Your goals should reflect your personal desires and values, not what others expect of you. Authentic goals are more likely to drive your commitment.

Action Steps:

1. Take out a notepad or open a document on your computer. Write down your goals, ensuring they meet the criteria above.

2. Visualize your success. Imagine how achieving these goals will improve your life, boost your self-confidence, and make you feel.

3. Share your goals with a supportive friend or family member who can encourage you along the way.

4. Break down your long-term goals into smaller, manageable milestones. This will make your journey less daunting.

Remember, setting clear goals is the foundation of your intermittent fasting journey. It's not just about the number on the scale; it's about reclaiming your health, vitality, and confidence. As you set your goals and commit to them, you're taking the first, crucial step towards a brighter and healthier future. The path may have its challenges, but your destination is worth every effort.

Choosing the Right Intermittent Fasting Method

So, you've decided to embrace intermittent fasting as a lifestyle choice, and you're ready to embark on a journey toward improved health and well-being. Congratulations on taking that first step! But now, you're faced with a crucial decision: Which intermittent fasting method is the right fit for you? The world of fasting comes with a variety of options, and selecting the one that aligns with your goals, lifestyle, and preferences is essential. In this chapter, we'll help you navigate the sea of choices and find the perfect fasting method that suits your needs.

Understanding Different Intermittent Fasting Methods:

Intermittent fasting isn't a one-size-fits-all approach. It offers flexibility, allowing you to choose a method that aligns with your daily routine, dietary preferences, and health objectives. Here's a brief overview of some common intermittent fasting methods:

1. 16/8 Method: This approach involves fasting for 16 hours and eating within an 8-hour window. For example, you might skip breakfast and only eat between noon and 8 p.m.

2. 5:2 Method: With this method, you eat normally for five days of the week and drastically reduce your calorie intake (around 500-600 calories) on the remaining two non-consecutive days.

3. Eat-Stop-Eat Method: In this approach, you fast for a full 24 hours once or twice a week. For example, you might start fasting after dinner and not eat again until the same time the next day.

4. Alternate-Day Fasting: As the name suggests, you alternate between fasting days and regular eating days. On fasting days, you consume minimal calories or none at all.

5. Warrior Diet: This method involves fasting for 20 hours and having one large meal in the evening, often within a 4-hour eating window.

Choosing Your Ideal Fasting Method:
Selecting the right method is a personal decision, and it should take into account various factors:

1.   **Lifestyle:** Consider your daily routine and commitments. Some methods may be more compatible with your schedule than others. If you have a demanding job or family responsibilities, a flexible method like 16/8 might be a good choice.

2. **Dietary Preferences:** Your preferred eating patterns and food choices matter. If you enjoy larger meals and don't mind occasional all-day fasts, the Eat-Stop-Eat method could be suitable. If you prefer smaller, more frequent meals, the 16/8 method might be a better fit.

3. **Health Goals:** Different methods may cater to specific health objectives. For weight loss, you might opt for a method that creates a calorie deficit, such as the 5:2 approach. If you aim to control blood sugar levels, you could consider the Warrior Diet.

4. **Tolerance and Adaptation:** Your body's response to fasting can influence your choice. Some people adapt more easily to certain methods, while others find them challenging. Experimentation and patience may be needed to discover what suits you best.

5. Consultation: If you have underlying health concerns, it's wise to consult with a healthcare professional or nutritionist before starting any fasting regimen. They can provide guidance on which method is safest and most effective for your situation.

Action Steps:

1. Take time to reflect on your daily routine, dietary preferences, and health goals.

2. Research the different intermittent fasting methods in more detail to gain a deeper understanding of how each works.

3. Consider starting with a less restrictive method, like the 16/8, and gradually progressing to more intense fasting methods as you become comfortable.

4. Keep a journal to track your progress and note how your chosen method makes you feel physically and mentally.

Remember, there's no one-size-fits-all answer when it comes to choosing the right intermittent fasting method. Your choice should be a reflection of your unique needs and aspirations.

Creating a Personalized Fasting Schedule

Now that you've chosen the intermittent fasting method that aligns with your lifestyle and goals, it's time to craft a personalized fasting schedule. Your schedule will dictate when you eat and when you abstain from food, and it's a crucial component of your intermittent fasting journey. In this chapter, we'll guide you through the process of creating a fasting schedule that optimally suits your needs and maximizes the benefits of your chosen method.

Understanding Fasting Windows:

Fasting windows are the periods during which you refrain from eating, and they vary depending on your selected method. It's essential to grasp the specifics of your fasting window to make your schedule work seamlessly.

1. 16/8 Method: In this approach, you fast for 16 hours and eat within an 8-hour window. Common schedules include skipping breakfast and consuming your meals between noon and 8 p.m.

2. 5:2 Method: On fasting days, you restrict your calorie intake to around 500-600 calories. The other five days are for normal eating. You can choose which days to fast based on your preferences.

3. Eat-Stop-Eat Method: You'll do one or two 24-hour fasts a week. For instance, you might fast from dinner one day to dinner the next day.

4. Alternate-Day Fasting: This method involves alternating between fasting days and regular eating days. On fasting days, you may consume minimal calories or none at all.

5. Warrior Diet: Fasting for 20 hours and having one large meal during a 4-hour eating window is characteristic of this method.

Personalizing Your Fasting Schedule:
Creating a fasting schedule that's personalized to your life involves making thoughtful decisions and adaptations:

1. Determine Your Eating Window: Choose the time frame during which you'll consume your meals. Make sure it suits your daily routine, work hours, and family commitments.

2. Flexibility: Be open to adjusting your schedule as needed. Life is unpredictable, and it's crucial to make your fasting plan adaptable.

3. Consistency: While flexibility is valuable, consistency is key for reaping the full benefits of intermittent fasting. Try to stick to your chosen schedule as closely as possible.

4. Meal Planning: Plan your meals to ensure they are balanced, nutritious, and aligned with your dietary preferences.

5. Hydration: Stay hydrated during your fasting periods with water, herbal teas, or black coffee. Adequate hydration is vital for your well-being.

6. Listen to Your Body: Pay attention to how your body responds to fasting. If a particular schedule makes you feel weak or overly hungry, consider adjusting it.

Action Steps:
1. Review your daily routine and commitments to determine the most practical fasting schedule for you.

2. Experiment with your chosen schedule for a few weeks, making note of how it affects your energy levels, hunger, and overall well-being.

3. Be prepared to adapt and fine-tune your schedule as you gain more experience with intermittent fasting.

4. Seek support from friends, family, or online communities to stay motivated and share experiences.

Creating a personalized fasting schedule is an essential aspect of your intermittent fasting journey. It's about aligning the method you've chosen with the rhythms of your life, making it a sustainable and enjoyable part of your daily routine. Remember, it's a journey of self-discovery, so be patient with yourself and embrace the process of finding what works best for you. Your personalized schedule will be the backbone of your intermittent fasting success.

Chapter 2

Understanding the Science Behind Intermittent Fasting

How Intermittent Fasting Affects Your Body

Intermittent fasting isn't just another diet trend; it's a scientifically grounded approach to transforming your health and well-being. In this chapter, we delve into the intricate workings of your body when you engage in intermittent fasting. Understanding the science behind it will not only reinforce your commitment but also empower you to make informed choices on your journey toward a healthier and more vibrant you.

The Basics of Fasting:

Fasting is a practice as old as humanity itself. Our ancestors often went without food for extended periods, not because they chose to but due to scarcity. This natural response to periods of food shortage is hardwired into our biology. Fasting is not a deprivation; it's an opportunity for your body to experience a break from digestion and tap into its innate healing mechanisms.

The Cellular Response:
When you begin fasting, your body undergoes a series of complex changes at the cellular level. Here's a glimpse of what happens:

1. Insulin Levels Drop: One of the primary changes is the significant drop in insulin levels. Insulin, a hormone produced in response to food consumption, facilitates the uptake of glucose by your cells. Lower insulin levels signal your body to start burning stored fat for energy.

2. Autophagy Activation: Fasting promotes a process called autophagy, which can be likened to a cellular cleanup crew. During autophagy, your cells break down and remove damaged or dysfunctional components, rejuvenating themselves in the process.

3. Ketosis:
In the absence of food, your body begins producing ketones, which are alternative energy sources derived from fat stores. This metabolic state is known as ketosis and is particularly associated with fat loss.

4. Hormonal Changes:
Fasting triggers a cascade of hormonal changes, including an increase in norepinephrine and human growth hormone (HGH). These hormones play essential roles in metabolism and fat burning.

Health Benefits of Intermittent Fasting:
Understanding the science behind intermittent fasting helps clarify the numerous health benefits it offers:

1. Weight Loss: Fasting promotes weight loss by creating a calorie deficit and accelerating fat metabolism.

2. Improved Insulin Sensitivity: Regular fasting can enhance your body's response to insulin, which is particularly beneficial for those at risk of or with type 2 diabetes.

3. Cellular Repair: Autophagy and the cellular cleanup process help repair and regenerate cells, potentially extending your lifespan and reducing the risk of diseases.

4. Heart Health: Intermittent fasting may lead to reduced risk factors for heart disease, such as lower blood pressure, improved cholesterol levels, and reduced inflammation.

5. Brain Health: Fasting may support brain health by enhancing brain-derived neurotrophic factor (BDNF), a protein associated with cognitive function, and reducing the risk of neurodegenerative diseases.

6. Longevity: While research is ongoing, some studies suggest that intermittent fasting might extend lifespan by promoting cellular resilience and health.

Action Steps:

1. Take a moment to reflect on how the science behind intermittent fasting aligns with your health goals.

2. Research further or consult with a healthcare professional if you have specific health concerns or conditions, to understand how intermittent fasting can benefit you.

3. Stay curious and open to learning more about the science behind fasting as you continue your journey. Knowledge is a powerful motivator.

Understanding the science behind intermittent fasting empowers you to make informed choices and motivates to stay committed. It's not a miracle cure, but rather a lifestyle that aligns with your body's natural processes, promoting health, longevity, and vitality. So, as you embark on your intermittent fasting journey, rest assured that you're engaging in a practice deeply rooted in the science of human biology.

Hormonal Changes and Metabolic Benefits

Behind the scenes of intermittent fasting's effectiveness lies a remarkable interplay of hormones and metabolic processes within your body. In this section, we'll explore the fascinating world of hormonal changes and metabolic benefits that make intermittent fasting such a powerful tool for improving your health, losing weight, and enhancing your overall well-being.

The Role of Insulin:

Insulin, often referred to as the body's "fat-storage" hormone, plays a pivotal role in the metabolic benefits of intermittent fasting. When you consume food, especially carbohydrates, your blood sugar levels rise, triggering the release of insulin. This hormone's primary function is to transport glucose into your cells for energy or storage. However, elevated insulin levels can hinder fat burning and promote fat storage.

The Fasting State:

During fasting, your insulin levels drop significantly, allowing your body to switch gears metabolically. This transition has several important consequences:

1. Enhanced Fat Utilization: With lower insulin levels, your body becomes more efficient at burning stored fat for energy. This can lead to weight loss and fat reduction.

2. Ketosis: In prolonged fasting or fasting methods like the ketogenic diet, your body enters a state of ketosis. Ketosis occurs when your liver produces ketones, which are an alternative energy source derived from fat. This metabolic shift can further accelerate fat burning.

3. Insulin Sensitivity: Regular intermittent fasting can improve your body's sensitivity to insulin. This means your cells become more receptive to glucose, resulting in better blood sugar control and reduced risk of type 2 diabetes.

Hormonal Changes:
Intermittent fasting prompts a series of hormonal changes, some of which include:

1. Norepinephrine: This hormone increases during fasting, leading to heightened alertness and energy. It also stimulates the release of stored energy, primarily in the form of fatty acids.

2. Human Growth Hormone (HGH): HGH levels surge during fasting, which has implications for muscle growth, fat metabolism, and overall body composition.

3. Adiponectin: Intermittent fasting can boost levels of adiponectin, a hormone that plays a role in fat breakdown and insulin sensitivity.

4. Ghrelin and Leptin: These hunger-regulating hormones experience shifts during fasting. Ghrelin, the "hunger hormone," increases before your eating window, signaling it's time to eat. Leptin, the "satiety hormone," decreases while fasting but rises when you eat, helping control your appetite.

Metabolic Benefits:
Understanding these hormonal changes leads to a range of metabolic benefits that are central to intermittent fasting:

1. Weight Loss: By increasing fat burning and creating a calorie deficit, intermittent fasting is a potent tool for weight loss.

2. Improved Insulin Sensitivity: Enhanced insulin sensitivity helps regulate blood sugar levels, reducing the risk of insulin resistance and type 2 diabetes.

3. Inflammation Reduction: Fasting can reduce chronic inflammation, a factor in various health issues, including heart disease, cancer, and autoimmune diseases.

4. Enhanced Brain Function: Improved brain-derived neurotrophic factor (BDNF) production during fasting supports cognitive function and may reduce the risk of neurodegenerative diseases.

5. Longevity: Research on animals suggests that intermittent fasting may promote longevity by enhancing cellular resilience and reducing age-related diseases.

Action Steps:
1. Reflect on how the hormonal changes and metabolic benefits of intermittent fasting align with your health goals.

2. Consider consulting with a healthcare professional or nutritionist to explore how intermittent fasting can be integrated into your wellness plan.

3. Stay engaged in your journey of learning and self-discovery. The more you understand the science behind intermittent fasting, the more effectively you can leverage it to improve your health and well-being.

Understanding the hormonal changes and metabolic benefits of intermittent fasting is essential to realizing the full potential of this lifestyle. It's not just about weight loss; it's about optimizing your body's natural mechanisms for better health, energy, and longevity. So, as you embrace the science behind intermittent fasting, you empower yourself to make informed choices that can lead to a healthier and more vibrant you.

Chapter 3

Preparing Your Body for Intermittent Fasting

Pre-Fasting Nutrition

As you embark on your intermittent fasting journey, it's crucial to prepare your body for the fasting periods to ensure a smooth and successful transition. This chapter focuses on the importance of pre-fasting nutrition, what you eat before entering a fasting window. By making thoughtful choices in this phase, you set the stage for a more comfortable and effective fasting experience. Let's dive into the essentials of pre-fasting nutrition and discover how the right choices can enhance your overall well-being.

Understanding Pre-Fasting Nutrition:
The goal of pre-fasting nutrition is to provide your body with the necessary nutrients to sustain energy levels during the fasting period. It's about making choices that promote satiety, stabilize blood sugar, and ease the transition into fasting.

Balancing Macronutrients:

1. Proteins: Include a moderate amount of lean protein in your pre-fasting meal. Protein helps maintain muscle mass and provides a lasting feeling of fullness. Sources like chicken, fish, tofu, or legumes are excellent choices.

2. Healthy Fats: Incorporate sources of healthy fats to support sustained energy. Avocados, nuts, seeds, and olive oil are examples of beneficial fats that can contribute to a sense of satisfaction.

3. Complex Carbohydrates: Opt for complex carbohydrates with a low glycemic index, such as whole grains, vegetables, and legumes. These release energy gradually, preventing rapid spikes and crashes in blood sugar levels.

Hydration:

1. Water: Stay well-hydrated, especially during the pre-fasting period. Adequate water intake helps curb hunger, supports digestion, and prepares your body for the upcoming fasting phase.

2. Electrolytes: Consider incorporating electrolyte-rich foods or drinks. Electrolytes play a crucial role in maintaining hydration, particularly important during fasting periods.

Meal Timing:

1. Consistency: Aim for consistency in meal timing, especially when following a regular fasting schedule. Establishing a routine helps regulate hunger and signals to your body that it's time to enter the fasting state.

2. Avoiding Excessive Caloric Surplus: While it's essential to nourish your body, avoid consuming excessive calories during pre-fasting meals. Overeating can lead to discomfort and negate some of the potential benefits of fasting.

Adapting to Pre-Fasting Nutrition:

1. Gradual Changes: If you're transitioning from a different eating pattern, consider making gradual changes to allow your body to adapt. Sudden, drastic alterations may cause digestive discomfort.

2. Listening to Your Body: Pay attention to how your body responds to different foods. Everyone is unique, so what works well for one person may not be the best choice for another. Tune into your body's signals and adjust accordingly.

Action Steps:

1. Plan Balanced Meals: Prioritize a balance of proteins, healthy fats, and complex carbohydrates in your pre-fasting meals.

2. Hydrate Adequately: Consciously consume water throughout the day to maintain hydration levels.

3. Mindful Eating: Practice mindful eating to foster awareness of your body's hunger and fullness cues.

4. Experiment and Adjust: Try various pre-fasting meals and observe how your body responds. Adjust your choices based on what makes you feel nourished and energized.

By paying attention to your pre-fasting nutrition, you lay a solid foundation for a successful intermittent fasting experience. The choices you make in this phase can influence your energy levels, mood, and overall well-being during fasting periods. So, as you prepare your body for intermittent fasting, remember that thoughtful nutrition is a key element in optimizing your health and embracing this transformative lifestyle.

Hydration and Electrolyte Balance

As you delve into the world of intermittent fasting, understanding the significance of hydration and electrolyte balance becomes paramount. Proper hydration not only supports your overall well-being but also plays a crucial role in making your fasting experience more comfortable and effective. This section explores the importance of staying hydrated and maintaining electrolyte balance, offering insights into how these factors contribute to a successful intermittent fasting journey.

The Importance of Hydration:

Hydration is a cornerstone of health, and its role is amplified during fasting periods. Water is essential for various bodily functions, including digestion, nutrient transport, temperature regulation, and the elimination of waste products. As you embark on intermittent fasting, here's why staying adequately hydrated is crucial:

1. Appetite Regulation: Drinking water can help curb hunger, making it a valuable tool during fasting windows. Sometimes, what we perceive as hunger is a signal of dehydration.

2. Energy Levels: Dehydration can lead to fatigue and decreased energy levels. By maintaining proper hydration, you support sustained energy throughout your fasting periods.

3. Digestive Health: Water is essential for digestion, aiding in the breakdown and absorption of nutrients. Proper hydration helps prevent constipation, a common concern during fasting.

4. Detoxification: Hydration supports the kidneys in filtering and eliminating toxins from the body. This is particularly relevant during fasting when the body may engage in autophagy, a process of cellular cleanup.

Electrolyte Balance:

Electrolytes are minerals with an electric charge, including sodium, potassium, calcium, magnesium, chloride, phosphate, and bicarbonate. Maintaining the right balance of electrolytes is crucial for numerous physiological functions, and during intermittent fasting, their role becomes even more pronounced:

1. Preventing Hyponatremia: While rare, excessive water intake without adequate electrolyte consumption can dilute sodium levels in the blood, leading to hyponatremia. Balancing water intake with electrolytes is essential.

2. Muscle Function: Electrolytes play a key role in muscle contraction and relaxation. An imbalance can contribute to muscle cramps and fatigue.

3. Nervous System Function: Sodium and potassium are critical for nerve impulse transmission. Proper electrolyte balance ensures the effective functioning of your nervous system.

4. Maintaining pH Balance: Electrolytes help regulate the body's pH level, ensuring that it remains within the optimal range for various biochemical processes.

Strategies for Hydration and Electrolyte Balance:
1. Water Intake: Consume an adequate amount of water throughout the day, especially during fasting periods. Aim for at least 8 glasses (64 ounces) daily, adjusting based on your individual needs and activity level.

2. Electrolyte-Rich Foods: Include foods rich in electrolytes in your diet. Bananas, oranges, leafy greens, nuts, seeds, and yogurt are excellent sources.

3. Supplementation: Consider electrolyte supplements, especially if you experience symptoms of imbalance such as muscle cramps or dizziness. Be cautious with supplements and consult with a healthcare professional if needed.

4. Hydration Schedule: Establish a hydration routine that aligns with your fasting schedule. Sip water consistently throughout the day and consider incorporating herbal teas or infused water for variety.

Action Steps:

1. Monitor Hydration Levels: Pay attention to your body's signals for thirst and ensure you're consistently hydrated.

2. Incorporate Electrolyte-Rich Foods: Include a variety of fruits, vegetables, and nuts that naturally provide electrolytes.

3. Experiment and Adjust: Find a balance that works for you. Experiment with different hydration and electrolyte strategies and adjust based on your body's response.

By prioritizing hydration and maintaining electrolyte balance, you enhance your body's resilience and support its functions during intermittent fasting. As you navigate this journey, remember that these simple yet crucial practices contribute not only to your physical well-being but also to the overall success and sustainability of your intermittent fasting lifestyle.

Meal Planning and Food Choices

Meal planning is the cornerstone of a successful intermittent fasting journey. Strategic food choices not only fuel your body during eating windows but also enhance the overall effectiveness of fasting periods. This section explores the importance of thoughtful meal planning and making mindful food choices to optimize your intermittent fasting experience.

The Role of Meal Planning:

Meal planning is more than a logistical task; it's a proactive approach to nourishing your body and achieving your health goals. Whether you're practicing intermittent fasting for weight loss, improved energy, or overall well-being, effective meal planning sets the stage for success. Here's why it matters:

1. Nutrient Balance: Planning meals allows you to ensure a well-rounded mix of macronutrients (proteins, fats, and carbohydrates) and micronutrients (vitamins and minerals). This balance is essential for overall health and sustained energy.

2. Portion Control: Intermittent fasting is not a license to overeat during eating windows. Meal planning helps you control portion sizes, preventing excessive calorie intake and promoting weight management.

3. Blood Sugar Regulation: Choosing nutrient-dense foods and spreading your meals strategically helps stabilize blood sugar levels. This is crucial for sustained energy and can contribute to better insulin sensitivity.

4. Satiety: Including foods rich in fiber, healthy fats, and proteins in your meal plan promotes a sense of fullness, reducing the likelihood of cravings or overeating.

Mindful Food Choices:
Making intentional and mindful food choices aligns with the principles of intermittent fasting and enhances its impact on your body. Consider the following guidelines:

1. Whole, Unprocessed Foods: Prioritize whole foods over processed alternatives. Fresh fruits, vegetables, lean proteins, whole grains, and healthy fats contribute to a nutrient-dense diet.

2. Lean Proteins: Incorporate lean protein sources such as poultry, fish, tofu, beans, and legumes. Protein supports muscle maintenance, aids in satiety, and can contribute to weight loss.

3. Healthy Fats: Include sources of healthy fats like avocados, nuts, seeds, and olive oil. These fats provide sustained energy and support various bodily functions.

4. Complex Carbohydrates: Opt for complex carbohydrates like whole grains, sweet potatoes, and legumes. These carbohydrates release energy gradually, preventing spikes and crashes in blood sugar levels.

5. Hydration: Integrate hydrating foods like water-rich fruits and vegetables into your meal plan. Proper hydration is essential for overall health and can also help control appetite.

6. Adapt to Your Preferences: Intermittent fasting is flexible, and your meal plan should align with your taste preferences. Experiment with different foods and recipes to find what works best for you.

Meal Timing and Composition:

1. Strategic Eating Windows: Plan your meals to coincide with your chosen eating windows during intermittent fasting. Consider the 16/8 method or other fasting approaches and adjust your meal timing accordingly.

2. Pre-Fasting Nutrition: Prioritize a balanced meal before entering a fasting period to ensure sustained energy and reduce the likelihood of hunger pangs.

3. Post-Fasting Nutrition: Break your fast with a balanced meal that includes a mix of macronutrients to replenish energy stores and support your body's needs.

Action Steps:

1. Weekly Meal Planning: Dedicate time each week to plan your meals. Consider your fasting schedule, lifestyle, and nutritional goals.

2. Grocery List: Create a shopping list based on your meal plan to streamline your grocery shopping and reduce the temptation to buy unnecessary items.

3. Preparation: Prepare ingredients in advance to make mealtime more convenient. This can include washing and chopping vegetables or pre-cooking proteins.

4. Experiment and Enjoy: Embrace variety and experiment with new recipes to keep your meals exciting. Enjoying your food is essential for long-term adherence to intermittent fasting.

By approaching intermittent fasting with a well-thought-out meal plan and mindful food choices, you not only support your health goals but also create a sustainable and enjoyable lifestyle. Remember that meal planning is a dynamic process, and as you progress on your journey, you'll discover the choices that work best for your body and preferences.

Chapter 4

Week-by-Week Guide to Intermittent Fasting

Week 1: The 16/8 Method

Welcome to the practical and transformative journey of intermittent fasting! This week-by-week guide is designed to ease you into the world of fasting, starting with the widely adopted 16/8 method. In Week 1, we'll explore the fundamentals of the 16/8 method, providing you with a structured approach to gradually integrate intermittent fasting into your routine.

Understanding the 16/8 Method:
The 16/8 method involves a daily fasting window of 16 hours, during which you abstain from food, followed by an 8-hour eating window. This approach is approachable for beginners and allows for flexibility in choosing when to begin and end your fasting and eating periods.

Day-by-Day Breakdown:

Day 1-2: Introduction and Preparation

- Familiarize yourself with the principles of the 16/8 method.
- Identify your preferred eating window within the 8-hour timeframe.
- Begin gradually adjusting your meal timing to align with the 16/8 schedule.

Day 3-4: Initial Fasting Periods

- Start with a 12-hour fasting window, extending it gradually each day.
- Focus on hydration during fasting periods to ease the adjustment.

Day 5-7: Full Implementation

- Begin the 16/8 method with a full 16-hour fasting window and an 8-hour eating window.
- Pay attention to hunger signals and experiment with nutrient-dense meals during your eating window.

Tips for Week 1:

1. Stay Hydrated: Drink water, herbal teas, or black coffee during fasting periods to stay hydrated and manage hunger.

2. Balanced Meals: Ensure your meals during the 8-hour eating window are balanced, incorporating proteins, healthy fats, and complex carbohydrates.

3. Mindful Eating: Practice mindful eating, savoring each bite and paying attention to your body's hunger and fullness cues.

4. Listen to Your Body: If you experience discomfort or extreme hunger, consider adjusting your eating window or experimenting with meal composition.

Reflection and Adjustment:

At the end of Week 1, take a moment to reflect on your experiences. How did your body respond to the 16/8 method? Did you encounter challenges, and if so, how did you overcome them? Use this reflection to make any necessary adjustments for the upcoming weeks.

Looking Ahead:

Congratulations on completing Week 1 of your intermittent fasting journey! As you move forward, remember that it's normal to encounter adjustments and challenges. The 16/8 method is just the beginning, and each week will bring new insights and experiences. Stay committed, stay curious, and embrace the process of discovering what works best for your unique body and lifestyle. In Week 2, we'll explore additional fasting methods to further customize your intermittent fasting journey. Keep up the excellent work!

Week 2: The 5:2 Method

Congratulations on completing Week 1 of your intermittent fasting journey! This week, we'll delve into the 5:2 method, offering you a new perspective on fasting. The 5:2 method involves regular eating for five days and restricting calorie intake on two non-consecutive days. Let's explore the principles of this method and guide you through a week of incorporating the 5:2 approach into your routine.

Understanding the 5:2 Method:

The 5:2 method introduces the concept of intermittent energy restriction. For five days, you'll eat normally, while on the remaining two days, you'll significantly reduce calorie intake, typically around 500-600 calories. The flexibility of choosing when to implement these fasting days adds a dynamic element to your intermittent fasting experience.

Day-by-Day Breakdown:

Day 1-2: Introduction and Preparation

- Familiarize yourself with the principles of the 5:2 method.
- Choose the two non-consecutive days for your reduced-calorie intake.

- Plan meals for the fasting days, focusing on nutrient-dense and satisfying options.

Day 3-4: Initial Implementation

- Begin with a regular eating day, focusing on balanced meals.
- Introduce the 5:2 method by reducing calorie intake on one fasting day. Monitor how your body responds.

Day 5-7: Full Implementation

- Follow the 5:2 method for the full two fasting days, keeping your calorie intake around 500-600 calories.
- On regular eating days, maintain a balanced and nutritious diet.

Tips for Week 2:

1. Fasting Day Nutrition: Opt for nutrient-dense foods on fasting days, incorporating vegetables, lean proteins, and healthy fats to maximize satiety.

2. Hydration: Stay well-hydrated, especially on fasting days. Water, herbal teas, and black coffee can be valuable companions during reduced-calorie periods.

3. Fasting Window: Choose fasting days strategically, considering your schedule and preferences. Some prefer consecutive days, while others space them apart.

4. Mindful Eating: Pay attention to your body's hunger and fullness cues on both regular and fasting days. Mindful eating enhances your connection with your body's signals.

Reflection and Adjustment:

At the end of Week 2, reflect on your experience with the 5:2 method. How did your body respond to reduced-calorie days? Did you find this method more or less manageable than the 16/8 method? Use this reflection to make any necessary adjustments as you progress on your intermittent fasting journey.

Looking Ahead:

You've successfully completed Week 2, embracing the 5:2 method and expanding your intermittent fasting toolkit. As you move forward, recognize the diversity of fasting methods and how each offers a unique approach to achieving your health goals. In Week 3, we'll explore another intermittent fasting method to further tailor your experience. Keep up the dedication and curiosity as you continue to discover the rhythm that best suits your body and lifestyle. Well done!

Week 3: The Eat-Stop-Eat Method

Congratulations on progressing to Week 3 of your intermittent fasting journey! This week, we'll explore the Eat-Stop-Eat method, a fasting approach that involves one or two 24-hour fasts per week. This method introduces a periodic and more extended fasting window, providing both physical and mental challenges. Let's delve into the principles of the Eat-Stop-Eat method and guide you through a week of incorporating this intermittent fasting technique.

Understanding the Eat-Stop-Eat Method:

The Eat-Stop-Eat method, popularized by Brad Pilon, entails a 24-hour fasting period once or twice a week. During this period, you abstain from food, allowing your body to experience an extended fasting state. This method emphasizes the importance of embracing occasional longer fasting windows for optimal health benefits.

Day-by-Day Breakdown:

Day 1-2: Introduction and Preparation

- Familiarise yourself with the principles of the Eat-Stop-Eat method.

- Choose one or two days in the week for your 24-hour fasts. Consider scheduling them on non-consecutive days.

Day 3-4: Initial Implementation

- Begin with a regular eating day, ensuring you have a satisfying and nutritious meal before entering the fasting period.
- Initiate a 24-hour fast, starting from your last meal of the day. Stay hydrated with water, herbal teas, and black coffee during the fasting period.

Day 5-7: Full Implementation

- Follow the Eat-Stop-Eat method with a complete 24-hour fast. Break your fast with a balanced meal after the fasting period.
- On regular eating days, maintain your usual balanced and nutrient-dense diet.

Tips for Week 3:

1. Fasting Day Nutrition: Prioritize nutrient-dense foods for your last meal before the fasting period. Include proteins, healthy fats, and complex carbohydrates for sustained energy.

2. Hydration: Stay well-hydrated during the fasting period. Consume water, herbal teas, and black coffee to support your body through the extended fast.

3. Mindful Reflection: Take moments during the fasting period to reflect on your body's signals and feelings. Notice any changes in energy levels, focus, or mood.

4. Adjust as Needed: If you find the 24-hour fast challenging initially, consider starting with a shorter fasting window and gradually extending it as you become more comfortable.

Reflection and Adjustment:

At the end of Week 3, reflect on your experience with the Eat-Stop-Eat method. How did your body respond to the 24-hour fasting periods? Did you find this approach manageable and sustainable? Use this reflection to make any necessary adjustments as you continue tailoring your intermittent fasting journey.

Looking Ahead:

You've now explored three different intermittent fasting methods, gaining a deeper understanding of how your body responds to various approaches. As you move forward, remember that flexibility and adaptation are key. In Week 4, we'll explore another fasting method, providing you with more tools to customize your intermittent fasting experience. Continue embracing the journey with curiosity and commitment, you're doing great!

Week 4: The Alternate-Day Fasting Method

Congratulations on reaching Week 4 of your intermittent fasting exploration! This week, we delve into the Alternate-Day Fasting (ADF) method, a more intensive approach that involves alternating between days of regular eating and days of either very low-calorie intake or complete fasting. This method challenges your body with alternating periods of nourishment and brief fasting, offering unique benefits. Let's explore the principles of the Alternate-Day Fasting method and guide you through a week of incorporating this intermittent fasting technique.

Understanding the Alternate-Day Fasting Method:
Alternate-day fasting involves cycling between days of unrestricted eating and days of either very low-calorie intake or complete fasting. This method can take various forms, allowing for flexibility in adjusting the level of caloric restriction on fasting days. It aims to create a significant calorie deficit, promoting weight loss and potential health benefits associated with intermittent fasting.

Day-by-Day Breakdown:

Day 1-2: Introduction and Preparation

- Familiarize yourself with the principles of Alternate-Day Fasting.
- Choose your approach: either complete fasting on alternate days or very low-calorie intake (around 500 calories) on fasting days.

Day 3-4: Initial Implementation

- Begin with a regular eating day, focusing on balanced and nutrient-dense meals.
- Introduce the Alternate-Day Fasting method by either fasting or consuming very low-calorie meals on the designated days.

Day 5-7: Full Implementation

- Follow the Alternate-Day Fasting method for the full week, alternating between regular eating days and fasting/low-calorie days.
- Pay attention to your body's response, energy levels, and any signs of discomfort.

Tips for Week 4:

1. Nutrient-Dense Eating: On regular eating days, prioritize nutrient-dense foods to ensure you meet your nutritional needs.

2. Hydration: Stay well-hydrated on fasting days. Consume water, herbal teas, and black coffee to support your body during periods of caloric restriction.

3. Meal Timing: Plan your meals strategically, especially on fasting days. Consider spreading smaller meals or snacks throughout the day to manage hunger.

4. Listen to Your Body: Pay close attention to how your body responds to alternating between regular eating and fasting days. Adjust your approach based on your comfort level and well-being.

Reflection and Adjustment:

At the end of Week 4, reflect on your experience with the Alternate-Day Fasting method. How did your body adapt to alternating between eating and fasting days? Did you find this approach manageable and sustainable? Use this reflection to make any necessary adjustments and gather insights for your ongoing intermittent fasting journey.

Looking Ahead:

You've now explored four different intermittent fasting methods, each offering a unique perspective on the relationship between eating and fasting. As you continue, remember that intermittent fasting is a highly individualized practice, and finding the method that aligns with your lifestyle and goals is key. In the coming weeks, you can experiment with variations or revisit methods that resonate most with you. Keep the curiosity alive, and embrace the evolving journey toward a healthier and more vibrant you!

Week 5: The Warrior Diet

Welcome to Week 5 of your intermittent fasting journey! This week, we'll explore the Warrior Diet, a method inspired by ancient warrior traditions that involves extended daily fasting and emphasizes the consumption of whole, nutrient-dense foods during a specific eating window. The Warrior Diet offers a unique approach to intermittent fasting, promoting both physical and mental resilience. Let's delve into the principles of the Warrior Diet and guide you through a week of incorporating this intermittent fasting technique.

Understanding the Warrior Diet:
The Warrior Diet is characterized by a 20-hour fasting period, during which you consume small amounts of raw fruits and vegetables. This is followed by a 4-hour eating window, typically in the evening, where you enjoy one large, balanced meal. The philosophy behind the Warrior Diet aligns with the idea that the body is more primed for digestion and absorption during the evening hours.

Day-by-Day Breakdown:
Day 1-2: Introduction and Preparation

- Familiarize yourself with the principles of the Warrior Diet.
- Choose a 4-hour eating window that aligns with your daily schedule, preferably in the evening.

Day 3-4: Initial Implementation

- Begin with a regular eating day, focusing on nutrient-dense foods.
- Initiate the Warrior Diet by consuming small amounts of raw fruits and vegetables during the 20-hour fasting period.

Day 5-7: Full Implementation

- Follow the Warrior Diet for the full week, emphasizing a single, large, balanced meal during the 4-hour eating window.
- Pay attention to your body's response, energy levels, and satisfaction with the eating pattern.

Tips for Week 5:

1. Balanced Evening Meal: During the 4-hour eating window, prioritize a well-balanced meal that includes proteins, healthy fats, and complex carbohydrates.

2. Hydration: Stay well-hydrated during the fasting period. Water, herbal teas, and black coffee can support your body through the extended fast.

3. Mindful Eating: Take time to savor and enjoy your evening meal mindfully. Appreciate the flavors and textures to enhance the overall dining experience.

4. Adapt as Needed: If you find the 20-hour fasting period challenging initially, consider adjusting the length or experimenting with the timing of your eating window.

Reflection and Adjustment:

At the end of Week 5, reflect on your experience with the Warrior Diet. How did your body respond to the extended fasting period and single, large evening meal? Did you find this approach to be sustainable and enjoyable? Use this reflection to make any necessary adjustments as you continue fine-tuning your intermittent fasting journey.

Looking Ahead:

You've now explored five diverse intermittent fasting methods, each offering a unique perspective on the relationship between fasting and eating. As you progress, consider incorporating elements from various methods or revisiting those that resonate most with you. The flexibility of intermittent fasting allows you to tailor the approach to your lifestyle and preferences. Continue with curiosity and dedication, knowing that your journey toward optimal well-being is a dynamic and evolving process. Well done!

Week 6: Combining Methods for Optimal Results

As you've progressed through your intermittent fasting journey, you've likely experienced the transformative power of this lifestyle. Now, in Week 6, we explore the concept of combining different intermittent fasting methods to amplify your results. This approach allows you to tailor your fasting routine to your unique preferences, goals, and lifestyle. By integrating various methods strategically, you can optimize your health, achieve weight management milestones, and foster long-term well-being.

Understanding the Synergy:

Combining intermittent fasting methods involves strategically alternating or overlapping different fasting windows throughout the week. This synergy can enhance the benefits of each method and address specific health and lifestyle goals. Here are some ways to consider combining methods for optimal results:

1. 16/8 + 5:2: Incorporate the 16/8 method on most days, restricting your eating to an 8-hour window. On two non-consecutive days, implement the 5:2 method by consuming a reduced calorie intake (around 500-600 calories).

2. Alternate-Day Fasting + Warrior Diet: Alternate between days of complete fasting and days of consuming one large meal in a 4-hour window. This combination can provide both the metabolic benefits of longer fasting periods and the simplicity of a compressed eating window.

3. Eat-Stop-Eat + 16/8: Integrate one or two 24-hour fasts during the week with the Eat-Stop-Eat method. On other days, follow the 16/8 approach for consistency and a sustainable routine.

Benefits of Combining Methods:
1. Enhanced Autophagy: Combining methods with longer fasting periods can promote more profound cellular cleanup through autophagy, supporting cellular repair and longevity.

2. Adaptation and Sustainability: The flexibility of combining methods allows for adaptation to different schedules and lifestyles. It can make intermittent fasting more sustainable in the long run.

3. Caloric Cycling: Alternating between methods introduces a form of caloric cycling, which can prevent metabolic adaptation and support ongoing weight loss.

4. Metabolic Flexibility: The combination of methods encourages your body to become metabolically flexible, adept at switching between using glucose and ketones for energy.

Creating Your Combined Plan:

1. Assess Your Goals: Clearly define your health and wellness goals. Whether it's weight loss, improved energy, or better metabolic health, understanding your objectives will guide your combined method choices.

2. Listen to Your Body: Pay attention to how your body responds to different fasting methods. Combining methods is a personal journey, and it's essential to adapt based on your unique needs and experiences.

3. Gradual Implementation: If you're new to combining methods, introduce changes gradually. Allow your body to adapt and observe how it responds before making further adjustments.

4. Consistency Matters: While combining methods offers flexibility, maintaining some level of consistency helps establish a routine that aligns with your lifestyle.

Action Steps:

1. Define Your Goals: Clarify your health and wellness objectives to tailor your combined intermittent fasting plan effectively.

2. Experiment with Combinations: Try different combinations of intermittent fasting methods over the week and observe how your body responds.

3. Assess Energy Levels: Monitor your energy levels, focus, and overall well-being to gauge the effectiveness of your combined approach.

4. Seek Professional Guidance: If needed, consult with a healthcare professional or nutritionist to ensure your combined plan aligns with your health profile.

As you enter Week 6 of your intermittent fasting journey, the exploration of combining methods offers a new dimension to your experience.

Chapter 5

Overcoming Challenges and Common Mistakes

Dealing with Hunger and Cravings

No journey is without its challenges, and embracing intermittent fasting is no exception. As you progress on this path toward better health, you might encounter moments of hunger and cravings. Understanding how to navigate these challenges is crucial for maintaining consistency and achieving success. In this chapter, we'll explore strategies to overcome hunger and cravings, empowering you to stay resilient on your intermittent fasting journey.

Understanding Hunger during Fasting:

Hunger is a natural and expected sensation, especially when you're adjusting to a new eating pattern. It's essential to differentiate between genuine physiological hunger and the conditioned response to regular mealtimes. Here's how to manage hunger effectively:

1. Stay Hydrated: Thirst can often be mistaken for hunger. Drink water throughout the day and during fasting periods to stay adequately hydrated.

2. Electrolyte Balance: Ensure you maintain a proper balance of electrolytes. Sometimes, imbalances can contribute to feelings of hunger or fatigue.

3. Gradual Adaptation: Your body may need time to adapt to a new eating schedule. Be patient and allow for a gradual adjustment period.

4. Nutrient-Rich Meals: Consume nutrient-dense meals during your eating windows to promote satiety and provide sustained energy.

Strategies for Overcoming Hunger:

1. Mindful Eating: Pay attention to your meals and savor each bite. Mindful eating helps you appreciate the flavors and textures, promoting a sense of satisfaction.

2. Fiber-Rich Foods: Include fiber-rich foods in your diet. They take longer to digest, helping you feel full for an extended period.

3. Protein Intake: Prioritize protein-rich foods. Protein has a high satiety factor and can contribute to a feeling of fullness.

4. Adjust Your Eating Window: If hunger is persistent, consider adjusting the timing of your eating window. Experiment to find a schedule that suits your body's natural rhythms.

Dealing with Cravings:

Cravings can be a common hurdle in intermittent fasting, often linked to psychological and emotional triggers. Here's how to manage cravings effectively:

1. Identify Triggers: Understand the root cause of your cravings. Are they tied to stress, emotions, or specific situations? Identifying triggers can help you address them more effectively.

2. Mindful Indulgence: If a craving persists, allow yourself a mindful indulgence. Consume a small portion of the desired food, savoring it without guilt. This can prevent feelings of deprivation.

3. Distract Yourself: Engage in activities that divert your attention from cravings. Whether it's going for a walk, practicing a hobby, or chatting with a friend, distraction can be a powerful tool.

4. Opt for Healthy Alternatives: If possible, choose healthier alternatives that satisfy your cravings without derailing your progress. For example, if you crave sweets, opt for a piece of fruit.

Action Steps:

1. Keep a Hunger Journal: Track your hunger levels throughout the day. This can help you identify patterns and make informed adjustments to your eating schedule.

2. Experiment with Meal Composition: Adjust the composition of your meals to find what keeps you feeling satisfied for longer periods.

3. Build a Support System: Share your intermittent fasting journey with friends or family. Having a support system can encourage during challenging times.

4. Mindful Practices: Incorporate mindfulness techniques, such as deep breathing or meditation, to manage stress and emotional triggers that contribute to cravings.

Conclusion:

Overcoming hunger and cravings is a natural part of the intermittent fasting journey. It's a process of self-discovery and learning to listen to your body's signals. By implementing these strategies and staying attuned to your needs, you can navigate these challenges with resilience, ensuring that hunger and cravings don't become roadblocks but rather stepping stones toward your health and wellness goals.

Staying Consistent with Your Fasting Routine

Consistency is the bedrock of success in any endeavor, and intermittent fasting is no exception. As you navigate the various methods and benefits of this lifestyle, maintaining a consistent fasting routine becomes crucial for long-term success. In this section, we'll explore strategies to help you stay steadfast on your intermittent fasting journey, ensuring that your commitment remains strong and your goals are within reach.

Understanding the Power of Consistency:
Consistency is the secret sauce that transforms intermittent fasting from a temporary practice to a sustainable lifestyle. It fosters routine, enables adaptation, and allows your body to reap the full benefits of fasting. Here's why consistency matters:

1. Metabolic Adaptation: Your body adapts to routines. Consistent fasting signals to your biological clock, optimizing metabolic processes and supporting the efficient use of energy.

2. Hormonal Balance: Regular fasting helps maintain hormonal balance, promoting stable insulin levels, enhanced growth hormone production, and other metabolic benefits.

3. Cognitive Reinforcement: Consistency reinforces the psychological aspects of fasting. It becomes a natural part of your routine, reducing decision fatigue and making adherence more manageable.

4. Sustainable Habits: Building consistent habits contributes to sustainability. Over time, intermittent fasting becomes second nature, woven seamlessly into your daily life.

Strategies for Maintaining Consistency:
1. Establish a Routine: Set a specific time for your fasting and eating windows, aligning them with your daily schedule. Consistency in timing helps regulate hunger and reinforces your body's internal clock.

2. Plan Your Meals: Prepare your meals in advance, especially during your eating windows. Having nutritious, balanced meals ready reduces the likelihood of straying from your fasting routine.

3. Use Technology: Leverage smartphone apps or reminders to track your fasting periods. Technology can serve as a helpful tool to stay accountable and maintain consistency.

4. Flexible Adherence: While routine is essential, be open to some flexibility. Life is dynamic, and occasional adjustments to your fasting schedule are natural. The key is to return to your routine promptly.

Building Mental Resilience:

1. Set Realistic Goals: Establish achievable milestones for your intermittent fasting journey. Realistic goals make consistency more attainable and encourage a positive mindset.

2. Celebrate Progress: Acknowledge and celebrate your successes along the way. Recognizing the positive outcomes of your efforts reinforces the value of consistency.

3. Mindful Reflection: Periodically reflect on your journey. Understand the impact of consistency on your well-being, energy levels, and overall health. This mindfulness reinforces your commitment.

4. Create a Support System: Share your intermittent fasting goals with friends, and family, or join online communities. A supportive network can encourage during challenging times.

Overcoming Setbacks:

1. Learn from Challenges: View setbacks as opportunities for learning rather than failures. Understand the factors that led to a deviation from your routine and use that knowledge to adjust and improve.

2. Adapt and Reassess: Life is dynamic, and circumstances change. If your initial fasting routine becomes challenging, be open to adapting it. Regularly reassess your goals and adjust your plan accordingly.

3. Avoid All-or-Nothing Thinking: Perfection is not the goal; consistency is. Avoid the trap of all-or-nothing thinking. If you miss a fasting period or indulge during an eating window, accept it, and commit to returning to your routine.

Action Steps:

1. Review Your Routine: Take a moment to assess your current intermittent fasting routine. Is it aligned with your lifestyle, goals, and preferences?

2. Implement Strategies: Choose one or two strategies to enhance your consistency. Whether it's setting a specific routine, planning meals, or using technology, implement changes that align with your needs.

3. Reflect on Progress: Reflect on how consistency has impacted your intermittent fasting journey. Acknowledge the positive changes and use them as motivation to continue.

4. Stay Resilient: Understand that challenges may arise, and setbacks are part of the journey. Stay resilient, learn from experiences, and stay committed to your health and well-being.

Consistency is the linchpin of success in intermittent fasting. It transforms the intermittent fasting journey from a short-term endeavor into a sustainable, transformative lifestyle. By implementing these strategies and fostering a mindset of perseverance, you'll not only stay consistent but also pave the way for lasting health benefits and well-being.

Avoiding Pitfalls and Misconceptions

Embarking on the intermittent fasting journey is a commendable step toward better health and well-being. However, like any lifestyle change, it comes with its share of pitfalls and misconceptions. Understanding these potential stumbling blocks is essential for navigating the intermittent fasting landscape successfully. In this section, we'll explore common pitfalls and misconceptions, providing insights on how to sidestep them and stay on the path to achieving your health goals.

Common Pitfalls:

1. Overeating During Eating Windows:

Pitfall: One common misconception is that intermittent fasting grants a free pass to indulge in excessive calories during eating windows, counteracting the benefits of fasting.

Avoidance Strategy: Practice mindful eating and focus on nutrient-dense, balanced meals. Be conscious of portion sizes to prevent overeating.

2. Neglecting Nutrient Quality:

Pitfall: Assuming that intermittent fasting alone guarantees health benefits can lead to neglecting the quality of the foods consumed during eating windows.

Avoidance Strategy: Prioritize nutrient-dense foods, including a variety of fruits, vegetables, lean proteins, and healthy fats, to support overall well-being.

3. Imbalance of Fasting and Feasting:

Pitfall: Some individuals may adopt an extreme approach, excessively fasting without considering the importance of balanced nutrition during eating windows.

Avoidance Strategy: Strive for a balanced approach, combining appropriate fasting methods with wholesome, well-rounded meals to support overall health.

4. Rigid Adherence to Fasting Windows:

Pitfall: Being overly rigid about fasting windows might lead to stress and disrupt the natural flow of daily life, making intermittent fasting less sustainable.

Avoidance Strategy: Be flexible with your fasting schedule, adapting it to your lifestyle. Allow for occasional adjustments without compromising your overall commitment.

Common Misconceptions:

1. Fasting Equals Starvation:

Misconception: Equating intermittent fasting with starvation might lead to fear or anxiety about the approach, deterring potential adopters.

Clarification: Intermittent fasting is a deliberate and controlled pattern of eating and fasting, distinct from starvation. It's about timing meals strategically, not depriving the body of essential nutrients.

2. One Size Fits All:

Misconception: Assuming that a single intermittent fasting method works universally for everyone overlooks individual variations in lifestyle, health conditions, and preferences.

Clarification: Intermittent fasting is highly adaptable. Experiment with different methods and customize your approach based on your unique needs and goals.

3. Quick Fix for Weight Loss:

Misconception: Expecting rapid weight loss without attention to overall lifestyle choices can lead to disappointment and frustration.

Clarification: While intermittent fasting supports weight loss, it's most effective when combined with a balanced diet, regular physical activity, and a holistic approach to health.

4. Ignoring Hydration:

Misconception: Neglecting hydration during fasting periods may be overlooked, assuming that only food intake matters.

Clarification: Staying adequately hydrated is crucial for overall well-being. Water, herbal teas, and other non-caloric beverages are essential components of successful intermittent fasting.

Action Steps:

1. Educate Yourself: Stay informed about the principles of intermittent fasting, its variations, and the science behind it. Knowledge is your best defense against misconceptions.

2. Prioritize Nutrition: Emphasize the importance of nutrient-dense, balanced meals during eating windows. Focus on the quality, not just the quantity, of the food you consume.

3. Experiment with Flexibility: Understand that intermittent fasting is not a one-size-fits-all approach.

Experiment with different methods and be open to adjusting your approach based on what works best for you.

4. Seek Professional Guidance: If you have specific health concerns or conditions, consult with a healthcare professional or a nutritionist to ensure that intermittent fasting aligns with your individual needs.

By being aware of common pitfalls and misconceptions, you empower yourself to make informed decisions on your intermittent fasting journey. It's not just about avoiding pitfalls but also about embracing a balanced, sustainable approach that aligns with your health goals and enhances your overall well-being.

However, like any lifestyle change, it comes with its share of pitfalls and misconceptions.

Chapter 6

Maximizing Your Results

Incorporating Exercise and Intermittent Fasting

As you continue your journey with intermittent fasting, unlocking the full spectrum of benefits involves synergizing this lifestyle with another crucial component: exercise. The combination of intermittent fasting and regular physical activity can amplify your results, promoting not only weight management but also overall health, strength, and vitality. In this chapter, we'll delve into the symbiotic relationship between exercise and intermittent fasting, offering insights on how to integrate both seamlessly for maximum impact.

Understanding the Synergy:
Intermittent fasting and exercise share common ground in promoting metabolic flexibility, optimizing hormonal balance, and supporting overall well-being. When these two components work in harmony, the results can be transformative:

1. Enhanced Fat Burning: Intermittent fasting already prompts your body to rely on stored fat for energy. When combined with exercise, particularly cardiovascular and strength training, you create an environment where fat burning is further optimized.

2. Muscle Preservation: Regular exercise, especially resistance training, helps preserve and build lean muscle mass. This becomes particularly crucial during fasting periods, as the body tends to utilize fat for energy while preserving muscle.

3. Improved Insulin Sensitivity: Both intermittent fasting and exercise independently contribute to improved insulin sensitivity. When combined, their effects are synergistic, creating a powerful strategy for managing blood sugar levels.

4. Increased Human Growth Hormone (HGH): Intermittent fasting triggers a rise in HGH levels, promoting muscle growth and fat metabolism. Exercise, especially high-intensity interval training (HIIT) and strength training, further stimulates the release of HGH.

Strategies for Integration:

1. Timing Your Workouts:

Strategy: Consider scheduling your workouts during or shortly before your eating windows. This allows you to replenish nutrients after exercise, supporting recovery.

2. Combining Cardio and Strength Training:

Strategy: Incorporate a mix of cardiovascular exercises (e.g., running, cycling) and strength training into your routine. This combination maximizes both fat-burning and muscle preservation.

3. Hydration and Electrolytes:

Strategy: Prioritize hydration, especially when exercising during fasting periods. Ensure adequate intake of electrolytes to support energy levels and prevent dehydration.

4. Post-Workout Nutrition:

Strategy: Consume a balanced meal or snack rich in protein and carbohydrates after your workout. This aids in muscle recovery and replenishes glycogen stores.

Tailoring Exercise to Your Fasting Schedule:

1. Training during Eating Windows:

Consideration: If your eating windows align with your workout times, ensure that you have a pre-workout meal or snack to provide the necessary energy.

2. Fasting-Adapted Workouts:

Consideration: If you prefer working out during fasting periods, focus on low to moderate-intensity activities or consider fasted cardio. Listen to your body and adjust the intensity as needed.

3. Adapting to Your Lifestyle:

Consideration: Choose exercises that align with your lifestyle and preferences. Whether it's morning yoga, an evening jog, or a lunchtime gym session, find what suits you best.

Monitoring Your Body's Signals:

1. Energy Levels:

Indicator: Pay attention to your energy levels during and after workouts. Adjust the intensity and timing of your exercises based on how your body responds.

2. Recovery:

Indicator: Assess your recovery after workouts. Adequate rest, sleep, and nutritional support are vital components of a successful exercise and intermittent fasting combination.

Action Steps:

1. Assess Your Current Routine: Evaluate your current exercise routine and intermittent fasting schedule. Identify areas where integration can be enhanced.

2. Set Realistic Goals: Establish realistic fitness goals that align with your intermittent fasting objectives. Whether it's weight loss, muscle gain, or overall well-being, clarity on your goals guides your approach.

3. Experiment and Adjust: Experiment with different types of exercises and timings to find what suits your body and lifestyle. Be open to adjustments based on your experiences.

4. Prioritize Recovery: Understand the importance of recovery in maximizing results. Ensure adequate rest, sleep, and proper nutrition to support your overall health and fitness journey.

By combining exercise and intermittent fasting strategically, you unlock a holistic approach to well-being. This synergy not only enhances physical fitness but also contributes to the comprehensive benefits of intermittent fasting. As you continue on this integrated path, remember that consistency, adaptability, and a mindful understanding of your body's signals are the keys to maximizing your results and achieving your health and fitness goals.

Tracking Your Progress

Embarking on the journey of intermittent fasting involves more than just a change in eating patterns, it's a holistic transformation that encompasses your entire well-being. Tracking your progress is a valuable tool that not only keeps you motivated but also provides insights into the positive changes occurring in your body and mind. In this section, we'll explore the importance of tracking, different methods to monitor your progress, and how this practice can enhance your overall intermittent fasting experience.

The Significance of Tracking:

Tracking your progress serves as a roadmap on your intermittent fasting journey. It offers several key benefits:

1. Motivation and Accountability:

Motivation: Regularly observing your achievements, no matter how small, serves as a powerful motivator to stay committed to your intermittent fasting goals.

Accountability: Tracking holds you accountable for your intentions, helping you identify areas for improvement and celebrate successes.

2. Identifying Patterns and Adjustments:

Patterns: Monitoring your progress allows you to identify patterns in your eating habits, energy levels, and overall well-being.

Adjustments: With data in hand, you can make informed adjustments to your fasting routine, exercise regimen, and overall lifestyle to optimize your results.

3. Celebrating Milestones:

Small Wins: Tracking enables you to celebrate small victories, fostering a positive mindset that contributes to long-term success.

Long-Term Goals: It keeps your long-term goals in focus, reminding you of the bigger picture and the progress you've made over time.

Methods of Tracking Progress:

1. Journaling:

How to: Maintain a journal where you record your daily fasting and eating times, meals, energy levels, and any observations or reflections.

Benefits: Journaling provides a comprehensive view of your habits, making it easier to identify patterns and areas for improvement.

2. Photographic Evidence:

How to: Take regular photos of yourself to visually document changes in your body composition over time.

Benefits: Visual evidence can be a powerful motivator and offers a tangible way to see the physical transformations occurring.

3. App and Technology Integration:

How to: Use dedicated intermittent fasting apps or health and fitness tracking apps to log fasting times, meals, exercise, and other relevant metrics.

Benefits: Apps often provide visual representations of your progress, making it easy to track trends and stay motivated.

4. Biometric Measurements:

How to: Monitor key biometric markers such as weight, body measurements, blood pressure, and blood sugar levels.

Benefits: Quantifiable data provides objective insights into your health and can guide adjustments to your intermittent fasting plan.

Establishing a Tracking Routine:

1. Define Key Metrics:

Identify: Determine the key metrics that align with your goals. Whether it's weight loss, improved energy levels, or enhanced fitness, clarity on your priorities guides your tracking.

2. Consistent Tracking:

Regular Updates: Make tracking a consistent part of your routine. Whether daily or weekly, regular updates provide a more accurate representation of your progress.

3. Reflect and Adjust:

Reflection: Periodically reflect on your tracked data. Assess patterns, milestones, and challenges to inform adjustments to your intermittent fasting and lifestyle approach.

4. Celebrate Achievements:

Acknowledge: Celebrate both small and significant achievements. Acknowledging your progress reinforces a positive mindset and fuels your motivation.

Action Steps:

1. Select Your Tracking Method:

Choose: Decide on the tracking method that aligns with your preferences and goals. Whether it's journaling, using an app, or a combination of methods, select what works for you.

2. Establish Tracking Habits:

Consistency: Make tracking a consistent habit. Set a specific time each day or week to update your records, ensuring you maintain an accurate and up-to-date reflection of your journey.

3. Set Realistic Goals:

Define: Clearly define your intermittent fasting goals and the metrics you'll track to measure progress. Set realistic milestones that contribute to your overall well-being.

4. Periodic Review and Adjustment:

Reflect: Periodically review your tracked data. Reflect on trends, achievements, and challenges.

Adjust: Use this reflection to make informed adjustments to your intermittent fasting routine, exercise plan, and lifestyle.

As you navigate the path of intermittent fasting, tracking your progress becomes a valuable companion on your journey. Embrace the practice with curiosity, use the insights gained to optimize your approach, and celebrate the evolving version of yourself that emerges through this transformative lifestyle.

Adjusting Your Fasting Plan as Needed

Flexibility is a cornerstone of sustainable health practices, and intermittent fasting is no exception. As you progress on your intermittent fasting journey, your body, lifestyle, and goals may evolve, necessitating adjustments to your fasting plan. This adaptability is key to maintaining a harmonious relationship with your well-being. In this section, we'll explore the importance of being attuned to your body's signals, signs that adjustments may be needed, and strategies for modifying your fasting plan as circumstances change.

Listening to Your Body:

Your body communicates its needs and responses, and attentive listening is vital for a successful intermittent fasting experience. Here's how to tune in:

1. Energy Levels:

Indicator: Persistent low energy levels or excessive fatigue may suggest that your current fasting schedule is impacting your overall vitality.

Adjustment: Consider tweaking the timing or duration of your fasting periods to align better with your natural energy rhythms.

2. Hunger and Satiety:

Indicator: Experiencing prolonged hunger or struggling with extreme cravings may indicate that your fasting windows need adjustment.

Adjustment: Experiment with altering the length or timing of your fasting periods to find a balance that suits your appetite and lifestyle.

3. Mood and Mental Clarity:

Indicator: Noticeable changes in mood, irritability, or difficulty concentrating might be linked to your fasting routine.

Adjustment: Fine-tune your fasting schedule to better support your mental well-being, considering factors like stress, sleep, and daily responsibilities.

4. Physical Performance:

Indicator: A decline in physical performance during workouts or difficulty recovering may signal that your current fasting plan is impacting your exercise routine.

Adjustment: Assess the timing of your workouts about your fasting periods, ensuring that you have sufficient energy for optimal performance.

Signs That Adjustments May Be Needed:

1. Plateau in Progress:

Sign: If you've reached a plateau in weight loss, muscle gain, or other health goals, it may be an indication that your body has adapted to your current fasting routine.

Adjustment: Introduce variations to your fasting schedule, such as altering the length or type of fasting, to challenge your body and stimulate progress.

2. Changes in Lifestyle:

Sign: Life circumstances, work schedules, or other lifestyle factors may shift, making your current fasting plan less practical or suitable.

Adjustment: Adapt your fasting routine to align with your evolving lifestyle, ensuring that it remains a sustainable and integral part of your daily life.

3. Health Concerns:

Sign: New health considerations or changes in medical conditions may warrant a reassessment of your fasting approach.

Adjustment: Consult with a healthcare professional to discuss how intermittent fasting can be modified to accommodate any health concerns or changes in your medical profile.

4. Stress and Sleep Patterns:

Sign: Increased stress levels or changes in sleep patterns can impact your body's response to fasting.

Adjustment: Prioritize stress management techniques and ensure adequate sleep. Adjust your fasting plan if needed to support your overall well-being.

Strategies for Adjustment:

1. Gradual Changes:

Approach: When making adjustments, implement changes gradually. Abrupt shifts may be more challenging for your body to adapt to.

Example: If extending fasting periods, add 15 minutes initially and observe how your body responds before making further adjustments.

2. Experimentation:

Approach: Intermittent fasting is a personal journey. Experiment with different fasting schedules, lengths, or methods to find what aligns best with your body and lifestyle.

Example: Try shifting your eating window earlier or later in the day to see how it influences your energy levels and hunger cues.

3. Regular Self-Assessment:

Approach: Periodically assess how your body is responding to your current fasting plan.

Example: Set aside time each month to reflect on your energy levels, mood, and progress toward your goals. Use this self-assessment to guide adjustments.

4. Professional Guidance:

Approach: If in doubt or if significant changes are needed, seek guidance from a healthcare professional or a nutritionist.

Example: Discuss any concerns or considerations with a professional to ensure that adjustments align with your health profile.

Action Steps:

1. Self-Reflection:

Assess: Reflect on your current intermittent fasting plan. Are you experiencing any signs that adjustments may be beneficial?

2. Identify Priorities:

Prioritize: Identify specific aspects of your well-being or goals that may benefit from adjustments, such as energy levels, appetite, or overall progress.

3. Experiment Responsibly:

Test: Experiment with modifications to your fasting routine. Start with small changes and observe how your body responds.

4. Seek Professional Input:

Consult: If needed, consult with a healthcare professional or a nutritionist to discuss potential adjustments, especially if health considerations are involved.

Adjusting your fasting plan is a natural and empowering aspect of the intermittent fasting journey. By staying attuned to your body, recognizing signs that adjustments may be needed, and implementing changes with care, you ensure that your intermittent fasting experience remains dynamic, adaptive, and supportive of your evolving well-being.

Adaptability is key to maintaining a harmonious relationship with your well-being.

Chapter 7

Living a Balanced and Healthy Lifestyle

Intermittent Fasting Beyond Weight Loss

Intermittent fasting is not just a diet; it's a lifestyle that extends beyond weight loss, embracing the holistic concept of health and well-being. As you navigate the various facets of this lifestyle, it's essential to recognize the broader impact it can have on your overall health. In this chapter, we'll explore the multifaceted benefits of intermittent fasting, emphasizing its role in promoting balance, vitality, and a sustainable approach to living a healthy life.

Holistic Well-Being:

Intermittent fasting transcends the scale, encompassing a spectrum of benefits that contribute to your holistic well-being. Beyond weight loss, here are key aspects to consider:

1. Metabolic Health:

Balance: Intermittent fasting supports metabolic health by regulating insulin levels, improving insulin sensitivity, and promoting efficient energy utilization.

Beyond Weight Loss: Even if weight loss is not a primary goal, maintaining a healthy metabolism is crucial for overall vitality and disease prevention.

2. Cellular Repair and Longevity:

Renewal: Fasting periods trigger cellular repair processes, including autophagy, which removes damaged cells and supports longevity.

Beyond Weight Loss: Embracing intermittent fasting fosters a cellular environment conducive to health and longevity, extending well beyond its impact on body weight.

3. Brain Health and Cognitive Function:

Clarity: Intermittent fasting may enhance brain health by promoting the production of brain-derived neurotrophic factor (BDNF), associated with improved cognitive function.

Beyond Weight Loss: A clear mind and heightened cognitive function contribute to a higher quality of life, influencing various aspects beyond physical weight management.

4. Inflammation Reduction:

Anti-Inflammatory: Intermittent fasting exhibits anti-inflammatory effects, potentially reducing the risk of chronic inflammatory conditions.

Beyond Weight Loss: Managing inflammation is integral to overall health, impacting aspects such as joint health, cardiovascular function, and overall disease prevention.

Balancing Health Priorities:

Living a balanced and healthy lifestyle involves recognizing and prioritizing various aspects of well-being. Intermittent fasting can be tailored to address specific health priorities:

1. Digestive Health:

Gut Balance: Intermittent fasting provides the digestive system with periods of rest, potentially supporting gut health and promoting a balanced microbiome.

Beyond Weight Loss: A healthy gut is fundamental to nutrient absorption, immune function, and overall digestive well-being.

2. Hormonal Balance:

Regulation: Intermittent fasting influences hormonal balance, including insulin, growth hormone, and cortisol.

Beyond Weight Loss: Hormonal equilibrium extends its positive effects to mood regulation, stress management, and reproductive health.

3. Heart Health:

Cardiovascular Support: Intermittent fasting may contribute to cardiovascular health by improving lipid profiles, and blood pressure, and reducing risk factors.

Beyond Weight Loss: A healthy heart is essential for sustained vitality, influencing energy levels, exercise capacity, and overall longevity.

4. Mindful Eating Habits:

Awareness: Intermittent fasting encourages mindful eating habits, fostering a conscious relationship with food.

Beyond Weight Loss: Cultivating mindful eating extends beyond calorie control, promoting a positive relationship with food and reducing the likelihood of emotional or stress-induced eating.

Sustainable Lifestyle Integration:

The sustainability of intermittent fasting lies in its adaptability to diverse lifestyles. As you embrace this lifestyle, consider the following:

1. Social and Cultural Considerations:

Flexibility: Intermittent fasting can be adapted to accommodate social events, cultural practices, and individual preferences.

Beyond Weight Loss: A flexible approach ensures that intermittent fasting seamlessly integrates into your life, supporting social connections and cultural experiences.

2. Physical Activity and Exercise:

Synergy: Intermittent fasting can be complemented by regular physical activity, creating a synergy that enhances overall health.

Beyond Weight Loss: Exercise becomes a joyful and integral part of life, contributing to cardiovascular health, muscular strength, and mental well-being.

3. Emotional Well-Being:

Balance: Intermittent fasting, when approached holistically, supports emotional well-being by reducing stress, promoting hormonal balance, and enhancing mood.

Beyond Weight Loss: Emotional balance contributes to resilience, mental clarity, and the ability to navigate life's challenges with grace.

4. Long-Term Sustainability:

Adaptability: Embrace intermittent fasting as a long-term lifestyle, allowing for adjustments as your goals, preferences, and circumstances evolve.

Beyond Weight Loss: A sustainable approach ensures that intermittent fasting remains a positive and enduring aspect of your journey toward optimal health.

Action Steps:

1. Reflect on Holistic Goals:

Consider: Reflect on the broader aspects of well-being that contribute to a balanced and healthy life. Identify areas beyond weight loss that align with your priorities.

2. Prioritize Well-Being:

Define: Clearly define your health priorities, encompassing physical, mental, and emotional well-being. Prioritize aspects that extend beyond the scale.

3. Tailor Intermittent Fasting:

Customize: Tailor your intermittent fasting approach to align with your holistic health goals. Consider adjustments that enhance various aspects of well-being.

4. Embrace Sustainable Practices:

Incorporate: Integrate intermittent fasting into your life as a sustainable and adaptable practice. Embrace a holistic approach that supports long-term well-being.

Living a balanced and healthy lifestyle with intermittent fasting involves recognizing the interconnectedness of various health factors. As you journey beyond weight loss, allow intermittent fasting to become a cornerstone of your well-being, supporting not only physical health but also mental clarity, emotional resilience, and a sustainable and joyful way of life.

Nutritional Guidelines for Non-Fasting Days

While intermittent fasting is characterized by designated fasting periods, the nutritional choices you make on non-fasting days are equally important for overall health and well-being. These days represent an opportunity to nourish your body with essential nutrients, support energy levels, and complement the benefits gained during fasting periods. In this section, we'll explore nutritional guidelines for non-fasting days, emphasizing a balanced and mindful approach to food choices.

Balanced Macronutrient Intake:

1. Protein:

Importance: Ensure an adequate intake of protein to support muscle repair, growth, and overall body function.

Sources: Include lean meats, poultry, fish, eggs, dairy products, legumes, and plant-based protein sources in your meals.

2. Carbohydrates:

Purpose: Carbohydrates provide energy for daily activities, and brain function, and support overall metabolic health.

Sources: Choose complex carbohydrates such as whole grains, fruits, vegetables, and legumes for sustained energy release.

3. Healthy Fats:

Role: Healthy fats are essential for nutrient absorption, hormone production, and overall cellular function.

Sources: Incorporate sources of healthy fats, including avocados, nuts, seeds, olive oil, and fatty fish, into your meals.

Nutrient-Dense Food Choices:

1. Colorful Vegetables and Fruits:

Vitamins and Minerals: Aim to include a variety of colorful vegetables and fruits to ensure a broad spectrum of vitamins, minerals, and antioxidants.

Fiber: The fiber content in fruits and vegetables supports digestion and helps maintain a feeling of fullness.

2. Whole Grains:

Nutrient-Rich: Opt for whole grains such as brown rice, quinoa, oats, and whole wheat, providing essential nutrients like fiber, vitamins, and minerals.

Satiety: Whole grains contribute to a sense of satiety and help regulate blood sugar levels.

3. Lean Protein Sources:

Satiety and Muscle Support: Prioritize lean protein sources for sustained satiety and to support muscle health.

Diversity: Incorporate a variety of proteins, including poultry, fish, beans, tofu, and yogurt, to ensure a diverse amino acid profile.

4. Dairy or Dairy Alternatives:

Calcium and Vitamin D: Include dairy products or fortified dairy alternatives to meet calcium and vitamin D needs for bone health.

Protein: Dairy also contributes protein and other essential nutrients.

Hydration:

1. Water:

Foundation: Hydration is crucial for overall health. Aim to drink an adequate amount of water throughout the day.

Meal Accompaniment: Drink water with meals to support digestion and help prevent dehydration.

2. Herbal Teas and Infusions:

Variety: Experiment with herbal teas and infusions to add variety to your fluid intake.

Antioxidants: Some herbal teas offer additional antioxidant benefits, contributing to overall well-being.

Mindful Eating Practices:

1. Portion Control:

Awareness: Be mindful of portion sizes to prevent overeating. Listen to your body's hunger and fullness cues.

Savoring: Take time to savor each bite, appreciating the flavors and textures of your meals.

2. Slow Eating:

Digestion: Eating slowly allows for better digestion and helps you recognize when you're comfortably satisfied.

Enjoyment: Enjoy the process of eating, focusing on the sensory experience of each meal.

3. Limit Processed Foods and Added Sugars:

Whole Foods: Prioritize whole, minimally processed foods over highly processed options.

Sugar Awareness: Limit added sugars and opt for natural sweeteners found in fruits when sweetness is desired.

Meal Timing and Frequency:

1. Regular Meals:

Consistency: Aim for regular meal times to establish a routine that supports metabolic health.

Balanced Intake: Consistent meals contribute to a balanced and even distribution of nutrients throughout the day.

2. Healthy Snacking:

Purposeful Snacks: If snacking, choose nutrient-dense options such as fresh fruits, vegetables with hummus, or a handful of nuts.

Energy Boost: Snacking can provide a quick energy boost between meals when chosen wisely.

Post-Exercise Nutrition:

1. Protein and Carbohydrates:

Timing: Consume a balanced post-exercise snack or meal containing both protein and carbohydrates to support recovery.

Hydration: Rehydrate adequately after exercise, especially if it involves sweating.

Action Steps:

1. Meal Planning:

Preparation: Plan balanced meals in advance to ensure a variety of nutrients and prevent reliance on convenience foods.

2. Grocery Shopping:

Diversity: Include a variety of fresh produce, lean proteins, whole grains, and healthy fats in your grocery list.

Read Labels: Pay attention to food labels to make informed choices about the nutritional content of packaged items.

3. Listen to Your Body:

Cues: Pay attention to your body's hunger and fullness cues. Eat when hungry and stop when satisfied.

4. Enjoy the Eating Experience:

Gratitude: Approach meals with gratitude, appreciating the nourishment they provide for your body.

Social Aspect: If possible, share meals with loved ones to enhance the social and emotional aspects of eating.

Incorporating these nutritional guidelines on non-fasting days complements the benefits of intermittent fasting, supporting your overall health and well-being. By embracing a balanced and mindful approach to nutrition, you contribute to a sustainable and nourishing lifestyle.

Long-Term Sustainability and Maintenance

Embarking on the journey of intermittent fasting is not just a short-term commitment; it's a lifestyle shift with the potential for profound and lasting effects on your health and well-being. Long-term sustainability and maintenance are crucial aspects of ensuring that the benefits you've gained remain integral to your daily life. In this section, we'll explore strategies to sustain intermittent fasting over the long term, adapt the practice to evolving needs, and foster a lifestyle that promotes enduring health.

Cultivating a Mindset for Longevity:

1. Viewing Intermittent Fasting as a Lifestyle:

Shift in Perspective: Embrace intermittent fasting as a sustainable lifestyle rather than a temporary solution.

Commitment to Well-Being: Consider how this approach contributes to your overall well-being, making it a permanent aspect of your health journey.

2. Setting Realistic Expectations:

Gradual Progress: Recognize that health and well-being are long-term endeavors. Set realistic expectations for progress, understanding that sustainable changes take time.

Celebrate Milestones: Celebrate small victories along the way, acknowledging the cumulative impact of consistent efforts.

Adapting to Life Changes:

1. Life Transitions and Adjustments:

Flexibility: Life is dynamic, and circumstances change. Be adaptable and open to adjusting your fasting routine to accommodate new responsibilities, schedules, or life stages.

Maintain Core Principles: While adjustments may be necessary, aim to maintain the core principles of intermittent fasting, such as mindful eating and time-restricted feeding.

2. Navigating Social Situations:

Communication: Effectively communicate your dietary choices to friends and family, helping them understand your commitment to health.

Flexibility in Social Settings: While maintaining your fasting routine, be flexible during social events, focusing on balance rather than rigid adherence.

Holistic Wellness Integration:

1. Comprehensive Health Focus:

Beyond Weight Loss: Continue to appreciate the holistic benefits of intermittent fasting, such as improved metabolic health, mental clarity, and overall vitality.

Regular Check-Ins: Periodically reassess your health goals and adjust your approach to ensure it aligns with your evolving priorities.

2. Integration with Other Healthy Practices:

Exercise Routine: Integrate intermittent fasting with a consistent exercise routine, creating a synergistic approach to overall health.

Stress Management: Prioritize stress management techniques, adequate sleep, and other components of holistic well-being that complement intermittent fasting.

Strategies for Long-Term Success:

1. Consistency and Routine:

Establish Habits: Create a routine that incorporates intermittent fasting seamlessly into your daily life.

Consistent Timing: Stick to consistent fasting and eating windows, reinforcing the predictability of your routine.

2. Regular Self-Assessment:

Reflect and Adjust: Periodically reflect on your experiences with intermittent fasting. Assess its impact on your well-being and make adjustments as needed.

Mindful Observation: Pay attention to how your body responds to the practice, incorporating feedback into your ongoing approach.

3. Educational Continuity:

Stay Informed: Stay abreast of research and information related to intermittent fasting, ensuring that your approach aligns with current knowledge.

Learning and Adapting: Be open to learning and adapting your practices based on new insights into nutrition, health, and well-being.

4. Community and Support:

Connect with Others: Engage with a community that shares your commitment to intermittent fasting. Share experiences, tips, and challenges, fostering a supportive environment.

Accountability Partners: Consider having an accountability partner who can provide encouragement and share in the journey.

Celebrating Non-Scale Victories:

1. Quality of Life Improvements:

Reflect on Non-Scale Achievements: Celebrate improvements in energy levels, mental clarity, and overall mood.

Enhanced Well-Being: Recognize how intermittent fasting contributes to your overall quality of life beyond numerical metrics.

2. Positive Relationship with Food:

Mindful Eating Practices: Continue to cultivate a positive and mindful relationship with food.

Enjoyment of Eating: Savor meals, appreciate the nourishment they provide, and derive enjoyment from the eating experience.

Action Steps:

1. Evaluate and Reflect:

Self-Assessment: Regularly assess your experiences with intermittent fasting. Reflect on the positive changes and areas for potential adjustment.

2. Adapt to Life Changes:

Flexibility: Be open to adapting your fasting routine to accommodate changes in your lifestyle, work, or personal circumstances.

3. Celebrate Progress:s

Non-Scale Achievements: Celebrate non-scale victories, acknowledging the holistic benefits of intermittent fasting on your well-being.

4. Community Engagement:

Connect: Engage with a community of individuals practicing intermittent fasting. Share insights, challenges, and successes to enhance the sense of support.

5. Educational Continuity:

Stay Informed: Stay informed about the latest research and information related to intermittent fasting, allowing your approach to evolve with updated knowledge.

Long-term sustainability with intermittent fasting is not just about maintaining a certain weight; it's about fostering enduring health, balance, and well-being. By adopting a mindset of longevity, adapting to life changes with flexibility, and integrating intermittent fasting into a holistic approach to wellness, you pave the way for a sustainable and fulfilling health journey.

Chapter 8

Troubleshooting and FAQs

Addressing Common Questions and Concerns

Embarking on the journey of intermittent fasting can bring about transformative changes, but like any lifestyle adjustment, it comes with questions and occasional challenges. In this chapter, we'll troubleshoot common concerns and provide answers to frequently asked questions, offering guidance to help you navigate your intermittent fasting experience with confidence and success.

Common Questions and Concerns:

1. I'm Not Seeing the Expected Results. What Should I Do?

Troubleshooting: Consider factors beyond weight loss, such as improved energy levels, mental clarity, and overall well-being. Evaluate your fasting routine, dietary choices, and lifestyle to identify potential areas for adjustment.

2. I Feel Hungry or Tired During Fasting Windows. How Can I Manage This?

Hydration: Ensure you're adequately hydrated, as dehydration can mimic hunger. Experiment with herbal teas, black coffee, or water during fasting periods. If fatigue persists, consider adjusting the timing or duration of your fasting windows.

3. Can I Exercise During Fasting Periods?

Exercise Timing: While light to moderate exercise is generally safe during fasting, some may prefer to schedule workouts during eating windows. Listen to your body, stay hydrated, and adjust your routine based on how you feel.

4. What Can I Eat or Drink During Fasting Periods?

Calorie-Free Options: Water, herbal teas, black coffee, and plain electrolyte drinks are typically allowed during fasting. Be mindful of additives that may trigger an insulin response.

5. I Have Digestive Issues. How Can I Address Them?

Fiber Intake: Ensure you're consuming an adequate amount of fiber from whole foods. Experiment with the timing of high-fiber meals and consider probiotic-rich foods to support gut health.

6. Is Intermittent Fasting Safe for Everyone?

Consultation with Professionals: Individuals with certain medical conditions or specific health concerns should consult with healthcare professionals before starting intermittent fasting. Pregnant or breastfeeding women and those with a history of eating disorders should approach intermittent fasting with caution.

7. What Can I Do If I Plateau in Weight Loss?

Variation in Routine: Introduce variations to your fasting routine, such as changing the duration or type of fasting. Evaluate your diet for hidden caloric intake and reassess portion sizes.

8. How Can I Manage Social Situations and Events While Fasting?

Communication: Communicate your dietary choices to friends and family. Plan your fasting and eating windows around social events, and be flexible without compromising your overall commitment.

9. Can Intermittent Fasting Help with Specific Health Conditions?

Research and Consultation: While some studies suggest benefits for conditions like insulin resistance and metabolic syndrome, individual responses vary. Consult with healthcare professionals to determine if intermittent fasting aligns with your health goals.

10. What if I Can't Maintain a Consistent Fasting Schedule?

Flexibility: Life is dynamic, and flexibility is key. If your schedule varies, adapt your fasting routine accordingly. Focus on consistency over perfection and make adjustments when needed.

Troubleshooting Strategies:

1. Periodic Self-Assessment:

Reflection: Regularly assess your physical and emotional well-being. Identify areas where adjustments may be needed and troubleshoot accordingly.

2. Gradual Adjustments:

Incremental Changes When troubleshooting, make adjustments gradually. Sudden shifts may be challenging to adapt to, both physically and mentally.

3. Professional Guidance:

Consultation: If encountering persistent challenges, consult healthcare professionals, nutritionists, or fitness experts. They can provide personalized advice based on your unique circumstances.

4. Community Support:

Sharing Experiences: Engage with the intermittent fasting community. Share your experiences and learn from others who may have faced similar challenges. Support and encouragement can be invaluable.

5. Mindful Observation:

Listening to Your Body: Pay attention to your body's signals. If a particular approach is not working, be open to trying different fasting methods or adjusting your eating habits.

Addressing FAQs:

1. Can I Drink Coffee or Tea During Fasting?

Generally Yes: Black coffee and herbal teas are typically allowed during fasting periods. Be cautious with added ingredients that may impact insulin levels.

2. How Long Does It Take to See Results?

Varies: Results vary among individuals. Some may experience changes within weeks, while others may take longer. Focus on the overall well-being improvements, not just the scale.

3. Can I Use Sweeteners During Fasting?

Limited Use: Some artificial sweeteners may be used in moderation, but be mindful of their potential impact on hunger and insulin response. Natural sweeteners like stevia are often preferred.

4. Should I Continue Intermittent Fasting If I Reach My Weight Loss Goals?

Personal Choice: Once weight loss goals are achieved, individuals can choose to continue intermittent fasting for its broader health benefits or transition to a maintenance phase with adjusted eating windows.

5. Is Intermittent Fasting Suitable for Athletes?

Adaptation: Athletes can adapt intermittent fasting to suit their training schedules. Timing eating windows around workouts and ensuring adequate nutrient intake are crucial for performance.

6. What Should I Do If I Overeat During Eating Windows?

Balance: Occasional overeating is normal. Balance your overall calorie intake and avoid compensatory restrictions. Focus on returning to a routine rather than dwelling on occasional indulgences.

Action Steps:

1. Self-Reflection:

Assessment: Regularly assess your experiences with intermittent fasting. Identify patterns, challenges, and successes to inform troubleshooting strategies.

2. Open Communication:

Community Engagement: Engage with the intermittent fasting community to share experiences and seek advice. Community support can offer valuable insights and motivation.

3. Professional Consultation:

Healthcare Guidance: Consult with healthcare professionals for personalized advice, especially if facing persistent challenges or having specific health concerns.

4. Mindful Adjustment:

Gradual Changes: When troubleshooting, make adjustments gradually. Listen to your body's responses and observe how changes impact your overall well-being.

Navigating intermittent fasting involves a learning process, and addressing questions and concerns is a natural part of the journey. By troubleshooting effectively, staying informed, and maintaining a mindset of adaptability, you can optimize your intermittent fasting experience for long-term success and well-being.

Handling Special Situations and Dietary Restrictions

Intermittent fasting is a flexible approach to nutrition, but its implementation may require consideration of special situations and dietary restrictions. Whether you're dealing with specific health conditions, adhering to cultural dietary practices, or navigating unique circumstances, this chapter will guide you in adapting intermittent fasting to meet your individual needs and goals.

Addressing Health Conditions:

1. Consultation with Healthcare Professionals:

Priority: Individuals with pre-existing health conditions or concerns should consult healthcare professionals before embarking on an intermittent fasting journey.

Personalized Guidance: Healthcare professionals can provide tailored advice, considering factors such as medications, metabolic health, and potential impacts on specific medical conditions.

2. Diabetes and Blood Sugar Management:

Monitoring: Individuals with diabetes should closely monitor blood sugar levels and work with healthcare providers to adjust medications as needed.

Type and Timing: Consideration of fasting methods, such as time-restricted feeding or modified fasting, may be necessary to align with diabetic management plans.

3. Pregnancy and Breastfeeding:

Caution: Pregnant or breastfeeding individuals should approach intermittent fasting with caution. Consult with healthcare professionals to ensure adequate nutrient intake for both maternal and fetal health.

Flexibility: Some may choose to adjust fasting windows or modify the approach based on individual needs and the advice of healthcare providers.

4. Eating Disorders and Mental Health:

Specialized Guidance: Individuals with a history of eating disorders or mental health concerns should seek specialized guidance from mental health professionals and nutritionists.

Mindful Approach: Intermittent fasting may not be suitable for everyone, and a mindful approach that prioritizes mental well-being is crucial.

Navigating Cultural and Religious Considerations:

1. Religious Fasting Practices:

Alignment: Some individuals may already practice religious fasting. Intermittent fasting can be aligned with these practices by adjusting eating windows or choosing fasting methods that complement religious requirements.

Consultation: Seek guidance from religious leaders or advisors to ensure that intermittent fasting aligns with religious fasting protocols.

2. Cultural Dietary Preferences:

Adaptability: Intermittent fasting is adaptable to various dietary preferences and restrictions.

Incorporate Traditional Foods: Consider incorporating traditional, culturally significant foods into your eating windows to maintain a connection with cultural dietary practices.

Adapting Intermittent Fasting to Dietary Restrictions:

1. Vegetarian and Vegan Lifestyles:

Plant-Based Protein Sources: Ensure an adequate intake of plant-based protein sources such as legumes, tofu, tempeh, and grains.

Diverse Nutrient Sources: Emphasize a variety of fruits, vegetables, nuts, and seeds to ensure a diverse nutrient profile.

2. Gluten-Free Diets:

Whole Food Emphasis: Prioritize naturally gluten-free whole foods, such as rice, quinoa, fruits, vegetables, and lean proteins.

Label Reading: Be vigilant in reading labels, as some processed and packaged foods may contain gluten.

3. Nut and Allergen Restrictions:

Substitute Safely: Individuals with nut or allergen restrictions can substitute alternative sources of healthy fats and proteins, such as seeds, coconut, or legumes.

Label Awareness: Read labels carefully to identify potential allergens in packaged foods.

4. Lactose Intolerance or Dairy-Free Diets:

Calcium Alternatives: Explore non-dairy sources of calcium, such as fortified plant milks, leafy greens, and tofu.

Protein Considerations: Choose alternative protein sources, including legumes, nuts, seeds, and plant-based protein supplements if needed.

Handling Special Situations:

1. Travel and Time Zone Changes:

Adjustment Period: Recognize that travel and time zone changes may require an adjustment period for your fasting routine.

Fluid Intake: Stay hydrated during travel, and be flexible with fasting windows to accommodate changes in daily schedules.

2. Shift Work and Irregular Schedules:

Adaptability: Intermittent fasting can be adapted to irregular schedules by adjusting fasting and eating windows accordingly.

Consistency: Strive for consistency in the timing of fasting and eating periods, even if work shifts vary.

3. Holidays and Special Occasions:

Flexibility: During holidays and special occasions, be flexible with your fasting routine while maintaining an overall balance.

Mindful Choices: Make mindful choices without feeling pressured to adhere strictly to fasting windows during festive periods.

Action Steps:

1. Healthcare Consultation:

Prioritization: Prioritize consultations with healthcare professionals, especially when dealing with health conditions, medications, or concerns about the impact of intermittent fasting.

2. Cultural and Religious Guidance:

Open Communication: Engage in open communication with religious or cultural advisors to ensure that intermittent fasting aligns with specific practices and requirements.

3. Adaptation to Dietary Restrictions:

Explore Options: Explore diverse food options within dietary restrictions, ensuring a nutrient-rich and varied intake.

Label Awareness: Stay informed about food labels, especially when navigating allergen restrictions or specific dietary preferences.

4. Mindful Approaches to Special Situations:

Flexibility: Embrace flexibility during special situations, such as travel, holidays, or irregular schedules, while maintaining an overall commitment to well-being.

Conclusion

As we draw the final pages of "The Beginner's Guide to Intermittent Fasting: A Step-by-Step Plan to Lose Weight, Improve Your Health, and Live Longer," it's evident that this journey is not just about shedding pounds but about transforming your relationship with food, health, and vitality. We've explored the foundations of intermittent fasting, delving into the intricacies of its various methods and understanding the profound impact it can have on your body and mind.

From the early chapters guiding you through the initiation of intermittent fasting, setting clear goals, and choosing the right method for your lifestyle, to the in-depth exploration of the science behind the process, hormonal changes, and metabolic benefits, each step has been carefully crafted to empower you with knowledge and actionable insights.

We've discussed the importance of personalized fasting schedules, pre-fasting nutrition, hydration, and electrolyte balance – all essential elements that contribute to a holistic approach to intermittent fasting. The subsequent chapters addressed challenges, common mistakes, and strategies for staying consistent, ensuring that your journey is not just a fleeting trend but a sustainable and rewarding lifestyle.

Throughout the pages, we recognized the significance of overcoming hurdles, embracing a positive mindset, and celebrating both scale and non-scale victories. We discussed troubleshooting strategies for common concerns, providing answers to frequently asked questions, and offering guidance to help you navigate potential roadblocks.

In the final chapters, we explored how intermittent fasting can harmoniously coexist with special situations, dietary restrictions, and unique circumstances, emphasizing adaptability and a personalized approach to suit diverse lifestyles.

As you close this book, remember that intermittent fasting is not a one-size-fits-all solution; it's a customizable framework that can evolve with you. It's a journey that extends beyond weight loss, reaching into the realms of improved metabolic health, increased energy, and longevity. It's a lifestyle that acknowledges the importance of balance, flexibility, and a positive relationship with food.

Your journey with intermittent fasting doesn't end here; it's a continuum, a path that you can tread with confidence armed with the knowledge, strategies, and motivation gathered from these pages. Whether you're a beginner taking the first steps or someone refining their approach, the principles of intermittent fasting can be your lifelong companion on the road to optimal health and well-being.

So, as you turn the last page, remember that this isn't the end, it's the beginning of a healthier, more empowered version of yourself. May your intermittent fasting journey be filled with resilience, joy, and the realization that you hold the keys to a vibrant and fulfilling future. Here's to embracing the limitless possibilities that lie ahead on your path to a healthier, happier life.